Bronx Rhapsody

poetry

Maria Meli

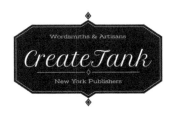

CreateTank Press

New York

CreateTank
2420 Bronx Park East, Suite 6C
Bronx, NY 10467
CreateTank on Facebook
www.facebook.com/mycreatetank
Email: createtankmedia@gmail.com

2018 CreateTank First Edition
Bronx Rhapsody
Copyright © 2018 by Maria Meli

Preface / Copyright © 2018 by Orlando Ferrand / Author photograph: Orlando Ferrand
Please, visit www.orlandoferrand.net for creative writing services and workshops

Book design: CreateTank / Cover design by Orlando Ferrand / Artwork by Maria Meli

To purchase a limited edition print of the artwork, limited edition book cover design posters, other limited edition artwork prints, and collectible-signed copies of *Bronx Rhapsody l*imited first edition hardcover, address createtankmedia@gmail.com

For information about exclusive discounts for bulk purchases, please email createtankmedia@gmail.com

Maria Meli is available for live events, recitals, lectures, and creative writing workshops. For more information or to book the artist and writer, please contact createtankmedia@gmail.com

Manufactured and printed in the United States of America

ISBN: 978-0-578-43045-4

Acknowledgments

For my father, Francisco Ciro Meli, who taught himself how to read and write with a second-grade education and read Walt Disney books to me as a child. He joined the Book of the Month Club so that he would always have books on hand. Thanks to him, I learned to appreciate how important it was to become a reader.

For my elementary school teachers, Ms. Lynch and Ms. Joyce, who gave me poetry books and novels during tumultuous times and sparked my love for reading and writing.

For Billy Collins, poet and professor of English at Lehman College, who noticed my talent before anybody else and wrote in one of my papers as a student that he "loved the street and spirituality" in my writing. Thanks to his encouragement, I continued.

For Charlie Vazquez, through whose diligence as director of the Writers Center at the Bronx Council on the Arts teachers were brought into our midst who creatively cajoled us into putting our thoughts down on paper.

For Orlando Ferrand, whose comment in the first class I ever took with him was to "dig deeper and write about what you have never told anyone." His insights, artistry, and fortitude have shaped the writer that I am today more so than anyone else.

For Robert F. Cohen, whose suggestions on restructuring my manuscript as well as his methodical copy edits have been crucial in achieving both linguistic cohesiveness and thematic clarity.

Editorial Team

Robert F. Cohen, Ph.D.

Orlando Ferrand

Preface by Orlando Ferrand

I dedicate this book to the good earth and all things green; to my Sicilian culture and its traditions; to my Grandma Teresa Meli and her sons, daughters, and their children; to my children, grandchildren, and great-grandchildren, who forced me to change.

Contents

AND THE BRONX WILL NEVER BE THE SAME

The words of *Bronx Rhapsody* move to the beat of Maria Meli's heart and the wrenching of her core. In her poems, one senses her relief and ecstasy for having been able to let go.

This second-generation Sicilian American takes us on a long journey, one that sings of her beginnings within the household of her immigrant family, enclosed by its traditions in its bucolic Bronx setting, and poignantly portrays her coming of age and her pilgrimage to adulthood. The trajectory embraces a luscious eight-decade life span from the time she was born in the years before World War II until the present.

But this volume of poetry is by no means a book of praise poems crafted after the dinner parties and rituals of warm Sicilian American families. Maria Meli allows us to bear witness to the challenges imposed upon her becoming a woman, all set against a poetic tapestry woven by a narrative of abuses and betrayals that include the Sturm und Drang of falling in and out of love and the joy only children can bring forth in the Boogie Down against the ever-changing backdrop of the City that Never Sleeps.

María Meli, just like her predecessors Anne Sexton, Audre Lorde, and Charles Bukowski, is a poet who is not afraid of exposing, denouncing, or uplifting humankind. She is both raw and sublime.

In her work, Meli questions assimilation against authenticity and condemns the hypocrisy of American politics and the proliferation of inequality, particularly amongst people of color, women, and the poor. Despite some scathingly ugly portrayals, her words, on the whole, reflect the poet's hope for all of us to rise above violence, erasure, poverty, and prejudice.

With such a spirit of optimism, Maria Meli also believes that we owe it to ourselves to feel, to name our own demons and dance with them because, in her view, it is precisely through the process of acceptance and forgiveness that starts within the self and radiates from us to our loved ones that we are genuinely able to open our hearts and embrace kindness and generosity as our daily mantra. Indeed, for Maria, achieving such a level of consciousness in our interactions with others can generate a kind of communal rebirth capable of restoring the dignity of all human life.

Orlando Ferrand

Bronx Rhapsody

Past, Present, Future

To youth I lost

the eternity of time

loose limbs

virginal blood

that seeped slow

into Gaia

pieces of myself

I had to hide

today I collide

with lost parts

and weep

wipe my snot and tears

on Sophia's hem of wisdom

I am weaning myself off grief

spiraling

a new fabric of being.

Numerology

Yesterday I was an eight

easily broken down by two or four

Put a blessing on myself

today I'm a nine

Mother Daughter and Divine

sacred trine is present

In my dream, I am Shaman

vibrating trees.

Grandma

Outdoors her green eyes glint gold in the rising sun

where she brushes her cascading white hair

effortlessly in front of the shack

that used to be the outhouse before plumbing

She winds and twirls her tresses

into a bun, secures it with long hair pins

on top of her head. Covers her hair

with a white scarf of authority and devotion

Legs like tree trunks, she embodied earth,

was my burdock, grappa, pomodoro, figs

She wore original crotchless underwear

a spread-spray maneuver gifted her pure nitrogen to the soil

(tales of Sicily memoried to us)

She knew herbs, cups, poultices,

removed *mala ochhio*

fasted, prayed novenas

And taught me how to hear the sounds,

see the visions

of her divinations

When we plucked chickens

she would say,

"*scald gaddina* to swell pores

feathers come out easy."

When she drew me close, her cotton printed dress

was my safety net. She smudged me with her white apron

wiping scrapes and tears.

I continue your way

and I've been told my green eyes glint gold

in the morning sun.

Melting Pot

America stole my language

In mandatory speech class

tried to smother me with

nylon, polyester, and sanitary napkins

Assimilation scoffed disquieted hands

telling their stories

said, "be a lady"

tried to Anglo me up from getting me down

My youthful warrior opposed

being a cultured hybrid

Forced to grow in whose pot of tradition?

Look for hard wood.

Chop, saw, and pile nearby *Granma's* cook stove

Scatter feed chickens, ducks, and pigeons

Don't let their water freeze

Wear gloves; fingers won't stick to water cans

Collect eggs

Feed rabbits, pigs, and goats

Eye animals for slaughter—Sunday dinner,

Christmas, Easter, too.

Repair coops to keep out cats and rats

Don't remove manure in winter; it's good

heat for the animals

Plant seeds, nurture them

in raised beds under old glass.

Summertime

gather fruit, vegetables,

flowers, herbs. Wash them, cook them, can them,

dry them, sell them. Press berries for wine,

soak peaches for brandy.

Your underwear; rub them together. Use washboard,

iron them. Scrub wooden steps, concrete floors. Set table,

clear table, wash dishes, dry dishes.

Walk dog, dress your brother, take him with you to the store.

Empty the garbage.

Free at last.

Edified physicality, consistency, courage

and between each breath

charm and terror

I identified with the aggressor

who taught violence

had loud opinions

would wreck objects

flesh and bone in one swipe

he starred in plays under kitchen lights

Grandma, Mom, Brother, and I

his vigilant audience

there was *Magia,* too

storytelling

music

dancing, games, and the art of food

we all suffered *dis-eases*

imbued by genetics

or behavior

in time

(it surely took a long time)

I learned to retain the positive

waive the negative and conjure up

posttraumatic growth in between.

hot blood Sunday into white panties

down familiar virgin thighs

onto hard mahogany pew

she bolts down church steps

embarrassed

runs against winter through swirling snow

that fashions her a maiden's crown

her heart bleats

beats faster nearing Paul's house

home

closed door behind her

she looks up to them

blurts out her newness

her flushed cheeks chastened

by her father's hand

and

there were other lessons about

not bathing, washing your hair, or touching plants

unclean she pauses

passing through tomorrows

swirling panties in cold water melting stains

snow piles in corners of window sill

house is warm with Sunday sauce

they call on her,

"Come down and set the table."

she was just a little girl who needed to pee

a house party crowded with relatives

piano keys being tickled, accordions squeezed

voices, contralto, staccato,

loud laughing

singing, gambling, dancing, fun

she was just a little girl in a narrow hallway

he stood close before her, reeking

of guinea stinkers and booze, reaching and groping

trying to mold her by squeezing

her supple youth

she was just a little girl

didn't scream, try to pivot, shift and leave

he, the aggressor,

she was just a little girl

a house with no eyes

a man with a little girl in a closet

she was there but not there, detached, indifferent

she only remembers her heart running so fast

Forty years later, her mother told me,

"I saw them

he, picking up his pants…"

perhaps she was for sale that day

for favors beyond her means or

maybe she was a gift for the company

she was just a little girl.

It was the '50s

Mambo Evolution

Titties bursting

We were wet and moist as dew

smelling of spunk and we wore rubbers

on our thumbs and index fingers,

MARWAY CARD FACTORY, BRONX USA

We flicked greeting cards

into envelopes, into boxes,

passing by on conveyor belts

If a perv boss was hot for you, you'd wind up

in any back room, away from assembly line,

working on specialty cards. There,

you had to learn to weave and spar

from feels, grabs, and the supreme

bowed "Head" routine, and

the incantation "touch it-touch it"

Lunchtime we spewed, he said, she said

flirted with *Fordham Baldies*—Blackie, in particular,

and they called us

"hot, teenage girls, factory workers, vulnerable."

We were vulnerable,

but on the crest of our

power.

Your curvaceous hills gave me speed, Mother.

I bicycled, sledded, ran down them fast.

Bronx River ran down them too,

streamed into the creek, the bay, and the sound.

Your hills were a lush place to hide

be coveted, fed by fruit

within arm's reach

from our mouths.

Your hills were black soil

and green everything,

now black and blue buried under asphalt

and concrete.

Changes

change is

still changing.

Your flatlands, Mother,

I used to see them from your hills,

salted green brown bush, humming.

Fertile waters filled with fish, eel,

oyster, crab, clams, pheasant, and duck.

Now uprooted,

unmoving under Co-Op City.

Silent under the Pelham Bay Dump.

Changes

change is

changing still.

Tonight,

under a crescent moon

driving down your hills,

changed, changing still

with a painful longing for family.

I cannot

will not

be who I was.

Intellect has eclipsed the Hero,

and Mother, Mother, how we have changed.

Ma

Pots and pans thrown at you. You, thrown down.

Misplaced in dad's mother's house.

Where was your place? Always in throes,

skittish, never a tear, a real wringing out.

A stoic dancer, city mouse in a country house.

Hated the itchy wool sweaters

you made me wear when ill to hold in heat.

Girdles to hold in my adolescent ass.

I believed you were a rose, Ma

whose thorns drip with blood

from my tattered hymen you didn't dare save.

I was never the ladylike child you needed.

Could never please you unless I was being you.

Being me, voices were raised in non-praise and degradation.

But I believe you're a rose, Ma

grown in potassium poor soul.

Stunted, struggling with your own pulse.

Peaceful essence close by but hard to reach.

A loving fragrance distilled in fear

bearing a silent burden,

your mother's, grandmother's, and sister's before you.

to mischief

messy magic

misbehaving

madness

saxophones

emptying political analysis

throwing out recipes

flicking

flexing

gliding

don't forget to undulate

all is well

we dream in code

keep it juicy.

I look for you, Sun, in this cold hard city

to shine on me,

I dodge monolithic mega shadows to be in your light

I follow you around clockwise

It saddens me to see you less

for darker skies and

winter's chill.

Forceful this eve

blue blasts

slapping me red

pushing on me

whips and snaps

whistling cool clues to my ears.

I ripple and weave

to play her off

and finally huddle

and give her my back.

Are you the wind of change?

I have been visited

welcomed sweet menses

flow

Bred to shed

mark me red

stain me ochre

Anoint me ancient ones.

Monoliths

rise

proclaiming

the dead.

A psychedelic shack across the track

Ray, Nina, Billie, Olatunji

wailing out the windows

dust dancing in hallways

you moving to the groove

breathing it all in

looking up at me from the stoop

me looking out the fifth-floor window

I knew you were the one, feline moves

voice, drumbeats, we became entangled

bone to muscle, pushing, pressing

out pain to the rhythm of our losses today

our anger tomorrow

we licked each other's wounds till our skin grew anew

where life cut us raw leaving beautiful scars

we were each other's habit

besides ruby port wine, junk and cannabis

you bathed me in warm water

your wet mouth drank my essence

we swallowed each other's desperation

through the night you palmed my vulva

suckled my breast

sang me to sleep after the loving

we were always high

bodies sensuous

serpents coupling

minds traveling between worlds

on a slow junk breath

in time, the cathedral we created

shrunk into a tomb

I had dreams

where you wouldn't walk

we received communion but not community

I left to gather

scattered seeds for a new spring

you accused me of fucking everyone

we started ripping each other apart

opening wounds we had already healed

it wasn't okay to drink each other's blood

I had to fly, my love

jonesed a long time without you

I still trip over our nights

Nina and Ray playing

the soundtrack of our lives

then the Raven flew and you ran away

your hospital records read

Psychotic Schizophrenic.

What the fuck was I?

Obsidian eyes smile, small centenarian body opens.

We give and take long strong close hugs

over espresso taste this and that we re-collect.

Used to be trees, their taste had story;

mulberry syrup, quince jam, peach brandy,

we knew how they got to our table.

Late summer smelled of swelled grapes, wet on wood.

The sun shone through a canopy of vines

for all seasons of our youth.

Granma's warm brown arms always around

family sang songs of assurance.

Our loose limbs leaped freely.

We laid low to sip from cold skipping streams

Jack in the Pulpit greeted us at springtime.

"Hey, you remember May Day, Mother's Day

you kids used to make wild flower bouquets

leave them on our doors and runaway?"

Rhythms of your voice lull me woman

native tongue beats of our past

paints panoramic view of our existence

and the body remembers.

"Small red ice small red ice"

the toddler says rapidly

from his mother's arms

on line outside the pizza shop

Waiting for ices

standing on the street I feel the heat

setting summer sun

hot on my calves

Brick Ovens of the Bronx

"Small red ice small red ice"

child's joy and innocence

oblivious to Italians

gesturing with passion

drunkard Irish woman

demeaning an Asian

he the new kid on the block

hip to its rhythms dances accordingly

Toddler's turn at the counter

his small voice rings out excitedly

"Small red ice small red ice,

one small cherry ice please."

Reminiscent Of A Bedtime

Little children get up in the middle of the night

to go pee or perhaps they've had a bad dream.

In our home, the bathroom light

was used as a nightlight

lighting their way.

Then, as the children became a little older

a light in the kitchen

close to the back door

was kept on

guiding them back home.

Bells are on the doors now

playing different melodies

depending on whose entering or exiting.

In the middle of the night or day

they can be heard

from upstairs, downstairs.

I usually can connect the rhythms

to the players;

the young men and women

coming and going.

P.S: Rest was always best

when they were all snug in their nest.

Lived with us since he was a kitten

as he got older he stayed outdoors more often.

He always came in on holidays.

Once, *Midnight* came home on Halloween and

stayed a while. His crooked ear,

gray hairs in his mane, begging for love.

It was cold out,

his hard fat body remembering its age stayed indoors.

He would come home to heal.

Spent a lot of time in the basement

being grumpy with the children.

They were vigorous and curious,

how *Midnight* used to be.

He continued to come and go.

After being away for a long time,

he returned on New Year's Eve, our holiday cat.

And then he left again. Or did he come back

that day in January never to be seen again?

Kids take your stuff.

When they're little,

they take all your time

get all your attention

kids get everything.

And they take your stuff when they've grown.

They take your BLS hat,

mess up your TV, camcorder,

eat up all your food,

and then leave.

Kids, when they return home to visit,

send this energy stream before them

this energy stream fills you with something you had

when they were little. It makes you cook, clean, bake, buy things

and get in touch with family members.

And then they go. Rooms and beds are vacant,

no babies in strollers, no high chairs.

There's silence, which absorbs loneliness

and tears for all that was and will never be again.

Your babies no more.

Their ghosts remain. You see their faces,

gestures, attitudes,

values, rhythms.

Their ghosts remain. You hear their voices.

Haven't read or opened your mail.

And you feel disoriented,

you've lost your current self, put it on hold.

You became Demeter.

Three days since they've been gone.

You've washed 6 loads of laundry

and began to put things back.

Made a pile of all the things you borrowed

to hold the grandchildren.

You start to re-member your now self.

Complain about this one's values,

that one's overprotectiveness.

But you understand why, and it's all OK.

You get on with your present self.

Reflect, give thanks for the experience of being Mother.

And keep on getting on with Artemis.

for Alysha

Grandchild's spirit

In child's

womb – belly – center – cauldron

once nested in Granma's

womb – belly – center – cauldron.

You've heard the drumming of our hearts.

You are

evolving – imprinted – patterned

Spirit of

air – wood – blood – water – earth.

All that's above – below – and center.

My grandchild,

you will arrive

with wisdom of the ages.

There was a time before the Greeks

that I can remember deep in the land.

I yearn for that time. Peace

a thousand years of peace.

It was a time of linking rather than ranking

partnership, instead of domination.

No centralized authority.

Palaces stood in communities,

and there were circular tombs.

Beauty surrounded the senses.

Equality and actualization were for all.

Art was unsigned.

Women were heralds in society.

Women and children

were not a commodity.

The rape

of women and children

was not glamorized, eroticized.

Crete 2000 BC

was centered around a King.

Communities became social hierarchies,

the people divided into

nobles, peasants, slaves

until this day.

We, women, have forgotten the gifts

that patriarchy has re-named.

Our autonomy is defined

as the need for Power.

Our blessedness looked upon

as witchcraft.

To meditate and dream is to be a heretic.

When we, women, bleed,

we are "polluted."

We have been orphaned

dis-membered by the death

of The Great Mother.

I remember summer time, long hot days. Early morning pulling in crab nets.

Ducks, pheasants, swans flying up like ribbons into the rising sun

because we spooked them. And how the creek was gently colored in hues

of pink and yellow. Sea grasses stood tall as we walked through them

cattails being the tallest.

I remember hanging on the block, leaning on the old Model T, biting into crab legs and

sucking on honeysuckle simultaneously. Our clothes were cotton

soft and soiled. The block was a dirt road. Our homes, gardens, and creeks

embroidered into the east side. Its west and south were woodlands, lush with

fruit trees, wild berries and a fresh water stream running away from the Bronx River,

singing. You could always hear it. On the north side were blocks of homes with

sidewalks and paved streets where Anglos lived. They called us Swamp Guineas, Dagos,

Wops.

In between them and us was a huge boulder with chokecherry trees growing

around it. A vantage point to see anyone coming toward us.

If they weren't friendly we would shoot our BB guns in their direction. I had a pump BB gun;

felt powerful with it. We shot at small game to eat and I'm ashamed to admit

birds for shooting practice.

I remember elderberries colored us magenta after cousins and I

squished them on each other.

And rope swings on horse chestnut trees whose roots drank

where fresh water stream and creek conjugated. It was the lowest point

of the woods, thick with skunk cabbage we used to wipe

our bottoms if we had to relieve ourselves. I remember playing Tarzan

 jumping off the rope swing onto an old mattress and yelling like

the wild man did all the way down. A snapping turtle as big as my chest lived there too,

he never snapped at us although we were constantly warned he would.

I remember playing Johnny on the Pony, Ringolevio,

I Declare War, Giant Steps, Cowboys and Indians, Cops and Robbers, Hide and Seek, and

shooting hoops through a barrel rim my cousin Giuseppe nailed on the light pole.

We had the teams; played stick ball, soft ball, baseball—our family was large.

My Aunt Vincenze who lived next door had twelve children

(she actually birthed thirteen; her oldest child died from consumption) and when her daughter Appolonia and her six children

visited on Sundays it was tribal.

I remember block parties after World War II. The sound of Jazz through horns,

husky vocals, piano, and nighttime. We made welcome home banners

with the names of our returning family members and hung them from tree to tree.

During the war, sirens would go off and we had to shut the lights and take cover.

There would be searchlights in the sky looking for enemy planes. My father,

an air raid warden, would put on a gas mask and go outside with other men

to patrol our neighborhood and keep families safe in the dark.

I remember dancing on stage at the Bronx Winter Garden to

"When Francis Dances with Me."

Holy gee. I'm as gay as can be, he takes me to dances 'cause

that's what I love, I fit in his arms just like a glove.

I learned tap, toe, and acrobatics.

My father sent me to dance school to make a lady out of me;

I was such a "Tom Boy"—whatever that means. I thought I was being authentic.

I remember timing how long my teenage lover and I would kiss.

White grapes hung above us behind the shed. Other couples would time us

for comparisons. We did it in lots of places, vine caves,

under the apple tree, in rock caves. He was fifteen I, eleven. Later

he fathered five of my six children.

I remember jarring tomatoes in the fall. Plunging chickens or pigeons

into boiling water, then plucking them—it was easier that way.

I remember mashing grapes and getting bit by bees and yellow jackets.

I remember my cousin Fidel skinning goats and rabbits; he was good at it.

Their skin would come off like a coat.

When Uncle Giacinto killed the pigs by slitting their throats

he would punch them so the blood would run out quicker. The men would drink it

and made blood sausage too. One time P.S. 97, the elementary school we attended,

had a field trip to our block to see our animals. We had goats, pigs, chickens, rabbits and

pigeons. They called us Swamp Guineas.

I remember sitting on the steps after a heavy rain reading and getting bit by fire ants.

I had red hot spots all over me. For all seasons

we spent a lot of time outdoors. I remember wildcats attacked our rabbit coops and while

cleaning a rabbit's wounds how he pissed all over me. I remember how we had to separate the

baby rabbits from the males because they would eat them. I remember *Nonna* sending me out

to pick plantain and clover for her poultices; chokecherries for wine.

The plantain and clover we gathered in wooden baskets with wire handles.

I would climb high in the trees with a few one-quart

aluminum canteens left over from the war tied around my waist and filled them. Two quarts

of chokecherries made a gallon of wine.

I remember playing hooky in first grade, hiding

behind Kruger's grocery store all day afraid someone would see me. I remember

stealing penny candies and comic books from Vinny's. We stole

outboard motors from Anglo yards, cigarettes from delivery trucks,

and sold them to the older guys. Got busted too in fifth grade

passing a note to my best friend Jr. Troiano as to where the cigarettes were stashed.

Our grandmothers beat us with a wooden spoon, not hard though. We found out that day

that our grandmothers came from Sicily together.

I remember smoking grape leaves and dinchers men dropped, drinking out of barrels.

At that time nobody locked their doors and just about everyone made booze. We would go into people's basements and wine cellars to get fucked up. I remember the first time

he said open your legs, bitch. Mom thought I got my period twice that month.

I remember Sundays getting dressed up in stiletto heels and black seamed stockings,

shoulder pads, tight skirts and sweaters with pointy bras and orange lipstick. Walking

to Pelham Bay Park, Loew's or Melba theatre. Hanging in the Astor Bar

smoking Chesterfields, sipping seven and seven, munching on French fries and dancing.

I was only fourteen.

I remember he tried to throw me in front of a car

'cause he thought I was pregnant. I remember a circle of men,

the light of the setting sun.

How I had to lay with the gang leader so that we wouldn't get jumped.

How it was never spoken of.

I remember praying

to the Blessed Mother all the time

for my period to come down.

How the soft green grass was swallowed in translation.

Our Stories took us here.

Right here,

to this place: South Bronx, USA.

Our stories do things.

They make sounds in the telling,

and re-telling.

And sounds move things, color them.

And those colors and sounds

are the weft and warp of our fabric.

They have power to conjure,

hold on to feeling good,

being blue, being black and blue.

Can someone else be dreaming us?

Let's name our illusions,

re-member ourselves even when

we are being dis-membered by fear,

shame, guilt, or as we stomp in joy,

moan in passion, and weep.

Can dreaming ourselves

be our timeless, internal dance?

When we step back

to view our looms

arms entwined, like warriors,

stronger silken threads

woven into patterns of

exuberance

will become the familial.

She had walked to my job; lived about 6 blocks away.

I was happy to see her. We were honest women

of 'questionable' morals. Had been around the block

many times, knocked down to rise again, sometimes

limping, in pursuit of our dreams.

We had met many years ago in the rooms of salvation.

What up

troubled mind?

I awoke to this guy mounting me

cock in hand—she sobbed. He came in through

the fire escape window. Warned

he would maim me if I screamed,

move or call the cops.

I didn't make a sound or fight.

He took all my money too.

We held on to each other

under a waterfall of quakes and tears.

Another woman child forcefully broken into.

It was the seventies, after all,

a time when rape tripled in New York

as the South Bronx burned. And AIDS was blooming,

traveling west.

"Squeal now, squeal like a pig!"

In 1972, *Deliverance* was showing that men

could also be forcefully broken into

out of jail.

I called a

rape hotline

heard a recording,

just a recording.

In our pain,

we received no directives.

Up on the roof sounded like a good idea

for solace and reprieve.

The sun was beaming.

Lying against a rooftop structure to soak it up,

we lifted our shirts

exposing our bellies,

heating Chi

pulsing Prana.

My mind began to cook. Come, it's time

to slay this dragon. We walked to

the local hospital's emergency room

where she was embraced with speed and empathy.

Finally, help for a woman child—A physical exam, blood, DNA tests.

From rapes in the seventies

many DNA tests taken were never read.

Through the healing balm of a feminist movement

rapes in New York have gone down.

But as of today,

rape kits have not been read yet,

some going back to the eighties.

What's a woman's status in this systemic folly?

When all was said and done,

a band aid was covering an abyss.

At the corner we hugged and began to part

back to our lives moving forward.

Hey, she said.

Sorry I upset you.

"Don't go," she sighs as the tiny bird flies

away from the ice-covered fire escape.

"Do you have a nest?"

A tattered blanket

shreds of her nest

warms her against winter's chill.

When the curtain of night

has fully risen

she searches

through the falling snow.

"Where's Papi?"

You are a rainbow

in a river full of sky

a voice inside

the voice inside

close to my bone

insisting

life's music

needs to be sung.

Ferry Point Park

Gray murky waters grasp

the shore, and meld.

Urban debris embarks plastics

within and without.

Plastics. Bags, diapers, dispensers

sheets and sheets of plastic,

on bough, feather, blade, and gill.

And those enjoying a

cooler summer breeze here

are too dulled to hear the gasping.

Portal

Sailing the forest, hidden steps rise

leading toward a solid wood door.

It opens easily into a room with

cathedral ceilings, high arched windows

from which diffused light enters.

Tints *olde* stone in pink hues.

Its quality is gossamer, undeveloped film

yet solid and strong. My essence,

blithesome, draped in soft gauze;

glides above ancient books

that lie open on stone ledges.

I shall return here often.

Your absence is my shadow

my body aches

in those places

you claimed for yourself.

Sometimes I dream you

out of the void, feel the weight

of your bones on our bed

you flee when I try to touch you

like dust in the afternoon sun.

I imagine you, an intimate breeze.

Your spirit is in the music of

Billy Joel, Marvin, and out to sea.

And in the concrete that you pounded

there's a curtain of fate billowing between us.

A common language

we probably no longer speak.

Silence betrays us.

Endings are beginnings,

gates of death and birth lay open.

I gather a harvest of swelled fruit,

witness that death has felled some

till birth or change.

Silence betrays us.

I carry fruit and seed to nest

savor, summon, covet

pick and sort toward the coming spring.

Happy New Year,

I shout silently.

Silence betrays us.

Sun journeys west

to the land of darkness

Earth lays to rest

with food and cover.

Mother sleeps

filled with seeds

she has drawn

deep inside her.

Death dwells

in the land of youth.

Through winter's dark time

She, cunt of the hillside,

awaits.

He, the cock of spring.

Old egg

Sol heats, penetrates

to your core

you yield steamy flora.

I

desire

      you

          dance

               for

          you

      with

you

          perineum

sphincter

          surrenders

      us

    free

In Between

Long smoke-filled afternoons

laced in lust under sheets

in ghetto wombs.

We grasp at rhapsodies,

to dance through life.

I've Dun Ravished You

The harmony of Southern Black

tickles me.

Halts me to savor it. I like the feel

of how it bounces and rocks me.

Off kilter, my thoughts liven with imagery.

I conjure up a valley green, enchanted.

I dressed sparse riding free on my black stallion.

You, perhaps a wandering warrior,

pull me down gently

like a laying on of hands.

You give much pleasure, I yield.

The valley is bewitched

balmy with flora and dew

a resonance of song birds.

We hinged, our rapture.

"Now that I've dun ravished you,"

was one of the lines in the last scene

before your exit.

A New Love

My heart and mind discussed you today

under a deep magenta sky at dusk.

Mind cold and calculating

reminded me of how you condemned yourself,

"dirty dog," "snake in the grass,"

excuses for being out of control.

I entertained the idea

that you may be the spider and I the fly.

Heart remembered your

wooly chest, soft lips, our laughter together.

Mind nudged.

Heart refusing to listen delved

just wished to remain uplifted.

Mind reminded me of pain endured.

Heart remembered too,

Cringed and closed you out.

Heart recalled the Prophet who spoke

of wheat needing to be threshed

mixed and kneaded before it is sustenance.

My heart thinks of you as sustenance

comes to you to feed.

My mind reminds me of parts of my whole that hunger too.

Will they be fed food they crave?

My spiritual teachings rang out,

"Emotions must be controlled

by the mind, Arjuna, on the battlefield of life.

Emotions are ruled by the senses."

Am I confusing heart with sense gratification?

Oh heart, help me now!

My heart opened

So, I went inside.

Missing You

Visit with me, my love

Come inside

Let us

Dance and weep

Lift our wings

Spread our tales

Above the trees

Roar and glide

Into the incoming waves

Which will return

Our sap to the wellspring.

Intermezzo

I love the way you reach

deep, up, inside of me,

going north.

And how I uncoil

going south,

getting down on it.

The afterglow lasts for days.

Magnetic sparks

have substance.

They carry me.

I lean on it.

I like it.

A Grandmother's Wish

I wish more fathers would be

at home with their families.

I wish America would stop persecuting

people of color, addicts, and the poor.

If only Big Daddy Prison Industries

fodder for the Upstate crowd

would not deny dignity to fatherless children

never forgiving their stories.

I wish America would stop redlining,

pulling rungs out of rehab, jobs, education

till our sons and daughters crawl on their bellies

on the same patch of concrete

in zip codes of no hope.

For how many generations?

If only equality were contagious.

There's no "liberty and justice for all."

There's just us. Unfortunately

most of us have baked a high moral pie

and think we're less oppressed.

I won't pledge allegiance!

Tuscany

I am a dazzling whirling wiggle giggle

moving backward in time.

Deep in this magenta forest

I be-dli-op with birds

chant at the moon

and suck persimmons.

Estrogen

Let's cavort the body's ripeness

sliding along

its crevices and mounds.

I am a ghost

ripped of flesh

and feelings

continually minimized

and reduced to

      "You."

By dusk you were gone
I walked the beach alone.

It revealed writings in the sand,
glacial rock coiffed with sea grass,
the color of spring, tidal music,
dancing footprints out to sea.

Today you and I
wore coats of sun and salt
dreamed islands, mansions,
Lenape Indians.

We played, Son
decades overdue.

I

A piece of my thumbnail breaks

I bite it off, spit it out

leaving DNA droppings somewhere.

Your coarse curls fall in clumps from your head

leaving more DNA here and there.

I wonder if you will live long enough

for them to grow again.

II

Our DNA is entwined, my brother.

Our souls rocked

in common matriarchal wombs.

We swam in the same embryonic pool.

You and I pushed our heels

down and out of a familiar slippery canal.

Shared domiciles; we were compromised and free for decades.

You and I, baby brother.

III

These days, bro, I hear less, can hardly smell;

find it hard to drive in the dark.

And you have lost most of your appetites for living.

You pace with consistent pain.

My pain lies in losing you

While the groom of crisis resurrects betrayals

In our family.

IV

You and I wore colors, bro,

red yellow purple black and blue.

Childhood bruises we tried to hide or

made up stories about. The exact colors we

gave to our children and they to theirs one way or another

along with the swing sway slam rhythms

of our beat downs. Notes passed forward.

V

You and I, bro,

developed hard body armor. Learned to strike

and hide to survive the balls pitched at us

vengeance hate revenge.

More DNA from our generational line?

Our home life was a war zone,

post war and depression era.

VI

When Dad died I didn't go to his wake or funeral

I was sick angry and hurt. We lived in a world of confusion.

He never apologized for our bloodied bodies.

When I asked how you were feeling about his death

You said, "I should've beat the shit out of him before he died."

We had a longing for love. And here we are today

You're dying; your children have drawn near to hold on

to what they never had and are losing again.

VII

We sit in epic.

I try to reason with you to make a last will and testament.

You say that magpie you've been living with for ten years

will take care of it and tell me what you want her to do.

I know this gluttonous woman will not comply.

Your children want it in writing too. You take it as an affront.

I remind you of Dad's legacy—he had no last will and testament.

VIII

Mom sold you and me out of our childhood home,

that incendiary house with no doors

where we bloomed and wilted under shameless eyes.

This woman has slid into the family wound and made it wider,

just like mom. They both knew not

how to sew, mend, or stitch.

IX

Your children keep slipping

falling down

into our blood.

DNA pouring from open wounds.

Leave your descendants something of yourself, my brother.

Time is of the essence.

It's moving and we can't stop it.

X

Say you're sorry It wasn't their fault

it was the only thing you knew.

Courage is being vulnerable, bro

it's the color of the heart.

We hold on to each other.

I feel his fleshless bones against my body.

"*Ci vuole coraggio*," I say

saddened that his children

will be betrayed and that another chorus

of this cry song is being sung

by our family.

FINI

Rest in Peace

In the chimney

I hear the wind howl

or is it I?

In the dark, shadows move

and breathe your pacing

in continuous pain

carrying

consciously, unconsciously

the betrayals of our ancestors

through relationships

I know

they were too heavy to escape.

Like a wolf I howl hoping to hear you respond.

Instead it's the storm of grief

I'm entertaining.

You're gone, left behind

is the bag of bones you became.

Your life will continue to blossom in me

the chubby toddler, awkward teenager

wild child on motorcycles, Doo-wop king

gardener, woodsman

mechanical wizard.

Tough guy guinea from the Boogie Down

uncanny psychic, a fighter.

You fought hard my brother

I will always honor the color of your heart,

coraggio. RIP my love.

I'm missing parts.

I'm frail and I whimper.

Grief wants me to hide

and only think of suffering.

She presses re-play

cancer, cancer,

cancer.

Hopeless without you

I flee to the woods, gardens

Places we shared.

You were trapped

in your own body. I wanted to share

your pain and fear.

Grief re-turns me

into a needy woman with fixed eyes,

not being able to see outside of myself.

Gradually, as I write, dance, shake off her scent and taste,

I re-claim my rituals

until we meet again.

I'm a "Swamp Guinea"

from those North-East Bronx marshlands

that history raped.

I'm from cousins called

Ciro, Giacinto, Appolonia

Vicenza and Carmine.

We fed goats, pigs

chickens, rabbits

harvested Bronx grapes.

I'm from underground cellars

smelling of wine wet on wood.

I'm from Sudan, Sicily

Sirocco Winds and West 4th Street.

Estuaries rivers streams

course through my veins

soil sand and low tides

ground me in place.

I come from tree whispers.

A line of women who wore

the blue cape of Madonna

scarlet letter of a harlot

who taught the ways of *La Strega*.

I come from the minds of

Madame Curie, Amelia Earhart

Dorotea Bucca, Tina Turner

and Nina Simone.

I'm from tomato plants, basilica

suspicious hearts of immigrants

gnarled hands that created

all the places I come from.

We have met Artemis

strong, lean, both of us,

predator and prey

Maternal to children,

animals, forests,

fiercely protecting them

Lying under the sky

with him or her,

you are the bridge to myself.

Maria Meli, a native New Yorker, earned a BS in Therapeutic Recreation at Lehman College and an MSW at Hunter College School of Social Work. She is an interdisciplinary artist who has worked extensively with intergenerational groups in both creative and therapeutic settings. Her poetry and essays have been featured in several anthologies such as *The Bronx Memoir Project Vol. 1* and *The Bronx Memoir Project Vol. 2*, and some have been performed in diverse venues in the U.S. Meli's insights into the human psyche are informed by her work as a performance artist, painter, clinician, Yoga teacher, single parent, mother, grandmother, great-grandmother and housewife.

CPSIA information can be obtained
at www.ICGtesting.com
Printed in the USA
BVHW010956140119
537773BV00020B/1540/P